HIV

FOR TEACHERS OF

Prevention

ELEMENTARY AND

Education

MIDDLE SCHOOL GRADES

Association for the Advancement of Health Education (AAHE)
in cooperation with
ETR Associates

This publication was completed with support from a cooperative agreement (#U62/CCU302780-04) between AAHE and the Division of Adolescent and School Health (DASH),Center for Chronic Disease Prevention and Health Promotion, Centers for Disease Control, Atlanta, Georgia.

1992

Written by Judith K. Scheer, EdS, CHES

©1992 by the Association for the Advancement of Health Education/American Alliance for Health, Physical Education, Recreation and Dance, 1900 Association Drive, Reston, VA 22091.

Developed by ETR Associates, P.O. Box 1830, Santa Cruz, CA 95061-1830.

Designed by Ann Smiley

Printed in the United States of America

ISBN 0-88314-517-0

Contents

Introduction

FOCUS

This preservice guide for HIV prevention education is designed to prepare university and college students to teach elementary and middle school children about the human immunodeficiency virus (HIV) and acquired immunodeficiency syndrome (AIDS). The guide provides students with knowledge, attitudes, and skills to effectively teach children about these topics. Students do not have to be medical experts on HIV, but they must have the skills and knowledge to answer children's questions. The guide also increases students' abilities to integrate HIV prevention education into the elementary and middle school curriculum. Through this guide, students can recognize and reduce their own fears and prejudices about HIV and AIDS.

TIME NEEDED

The time needed to present the material in this guide will depend upon a variety of factors, such as the students' knowledge of HIV and AIDS content, their knowledge of methods and resources, their skill in responding to children's questions, their degree of comfort with sensitive topics, and the amount of time available. However, it is suggested that at least three classroom hours be allocated to the material.

Students are asked to do outside reading before class and to complete an assignment after the material has been presented. It is highly recommended that the students receive basic HIV and AIDS information before the class by reading from the suggested list of resources found in the appendix. This guide includes excerpts from and makes reference to the publication *"Does AIDS Hurt?"* by Quackenbush and Villarreal (ETR Associates, 1988). This publication is an excellent resource for elementary HIV and AIDS prevention education. A video that provides accurate information is also recommended.

ORGANIZATION

The first chapter of this guide encourages university or college students to explore their feelings, attitudes, and prejudices about HIV prevention education. Chapter 2 provides an overview of the scope and sequence of HIV prevention education and addresses considerations for these programs.

Appropriately responding to children's questions may be the greatest single concern of future teachers. We can prepare students to handle children's questions by providing a strong knowledge base. We must also teach them how to uncover the true meaning of a child's question and respond to it with sensitivity. The response must be appropriate for the child's developmental level, reflect parent and community values, and maintain school policies and guidelines. Chapter 3 provides suggested guidelines and practice exercises for responding to questions.

Modeling classroom activities is useful and effective in enhancing learning opportunities. Appropriate teaching strategies are presented in Chapters 4 and 5. Chapter 4 focuses on identifying appropriate places in the early elementary curriculum for children to express their HIV-related concerns or fears. Students can learn to assess the level of concern among children and provide reassurance, correct misinformation, and make appropriate referrals for children with special concerns. In Chapter 5 students learn effective methods for addressing controversial topics. They should be encouraged to use the class activities to define what the new material means to them both *personally* and *professionally*.

Chapter 6 invites students to reexamine their personal attitudes, concerns, and prejudices about HIV prevention education. Students are required to create appropriate HIV classroom activities and to respond to potential questions from children.

Handouts, transparency masters, and resources follow each of the chapters.

ASSUMPTIONS

Because we have made certain assumptions in this guide, professors will need to adapt the material to fit the needs of their students. We have assumed that students have:

1. adequate background in learning theory, developmental stages of learning, social learning theory, cognitive-behavioral theory, and skills-based instruction
2. skills in teaching risk-reducing behaviors, such as decision making, communication, refusal skills, and problem solving

3. training in developing, locating, selecting, and using developmentally appropriate health education resources
4. skill in selecting and using culturally sensitive activities and materials
5. been taught how to keep their own attitudes, prejudices, and values from interfering with their role in supporting community and parental values
6. learned the importance of working with parent and community representatives to develop guidelines where none exist and how to enhance parent-child communication, supporting parents as primary values educators of the children
7. basic HIV and AIDS knowledge, gained by reading from the suggested selections in the resource list found in the appendix or other appropriate media or publications.

SCHOOL POLICIES ABOUT HIV PREVENTION EDUCATION

Students should be aware that most school districts have adopted policies and strategies for implementing HIV prevention education. Local school boards of education have the ultimate control in approving the curriculum within the context of state laws. Teachers must follow the approved HIV prevention guidelines when teaching HIV prevention education.

OBJECTIVES

Chapter 1 ◆ Assessing Personal Feelings About HIV Prevention Education
- Students analyze how personal feelings about HIV prevention education might affect their performance as classroom teachers.

Chapter 2 ◆ HIV Prevention Education: Scope and Sequence
- Students explain the function of HIV-specific and HIV-related content within an effective HIV prevention education program.
- Students describe how HIV prevention education fits into the elementary curriculum.
- Students describe how HIV prevention education fits into the concept of comprehensive school health education.

Chapter 3 ◆ *Responding to Children's Questions*
- Students compose an appropriate response to a child's question about HIV or AIDS.
- Students describe guidelines for formulating an appropriate response to a child's question.

Chapter 4 ◆ *Methods for Early Elementary Grades*
- Students describe the purpose of the Centers for Disease Control's *Guidelines for Effective School Health Education to Prevent the Spread of AIDS.*
- Students describe and create developmentally appropriate learning opportunities for early elementary school children.

Chapter 5 ◆ *Methods for Late Elementary/Middle School Grades*
- Students correlate developmental characteristics of children in the fourth through eighth grades with the essential information for HIV prevention education.
- Students describe appropriate strategies to teach children in upper elementary grades about HIV and AIDS.

Chapter 6 ◆ *Reassessing Personal Feelings and Staying Informed*
- Students describe the importance of a positive attitude toward HIV prevention education in the elementary and middle school grades.
- Students identify reliable sources of current information on HIV and AIDS.
- Students design an appropriate strategy for presenting HIV-specific information to elementary and middle school students (grades kindergarten through eighth).

MATERIALS NEEDED

Suggested activities and materials are appropriate at different grade levels. Some materials are appropriate for early elementary grades (kindergarten through third grade), while others are appropriate for late elementary/middle school grades (fourth through eighth grade). Information, activities, and materials must be age-appropriate.

General: Selected background reading (see **Essential Readings** in the appendix)
Overhead projector and screen
Transparency marker

Chalkboard

Chalk

Chapter 1 ◆ Assessing Personal Feelings About HIV Prevention Education

Handout: **Why Elementary/Middle School Teachers Might Choose *Not* to Teach About HIV and AIDS** (one for each student)

Chapter 2 ◆ HIV Prevention Education: Scope and Sequence

Transparencies: **Purpose of HIV Prevention Education and Health Framework**

Overlay A: **HIV:Related Content**

Overlay B: **HIV:Specific Content**

Resource: **Health Framework** (illustration of completed transparency)

Handout: **Sample Content Outline** (one for each student)

Handout: **Cultural Sensitivity for HIV Prevention Educators**

Chapter 3 ◆ Responding to Children's Questions

Transparency: **Question**

Overlay A: **Assess**

Resource: ***Real* Question** (illustration of completed transparency)

Chapter 4 ◆ Methods for Early Elementary Grades

Transparency: **Consultants for CDC Guidelines**

Handout: **CDC Recommendations for HIV: Related Information Provided in Early Elementary Grades** (one for each student)

Supplies: One small container of glitter

Study prints, magazine or coloring book pictures, puppets, or books illustrating health helpers

Eight 9-inch round balloons

Dark, wide permanent marker (for writing on balloons)

Pillowcase or white kitchen trash bag labeled WORRIES

Straight pin

Chapter 5 ◆ Methods for Late Elementary/Middle School Grades

Handout: **CDC Recommendations for HIV:Related Information Provided in Late Elementary/Middle School Grades** (one for each student)

Supplies: Tennis ball

Golf ball

Miniature marshmallow

Large plastic egg (such as L'eggs egg) that splits into halves

Ten to fifteen small marshmallows

Two clear, plastic bottles (juice bottles, tennis ball cans, or peanut butter jars) without labels, one half-filled with pale green water and the other half-filled with dark red water

Tape

Two pencils

Two small toys

Large see-through baster

Rag

Ten large pictures of men and women from various age and racial groups; include pictures of individuals living in city, suburban, and rural environments

Chapter 6 ◆ *Reassessing Personal Feelings and Staying Informed*

Handout: **Why Elementary/Middle School Teachers Might Choose *Not* to Teach About HIV and AIDS** (completed by each student in Chapter 1)

Handout: **HIV Prevention Assignment** (one for each student)

CHAPTER 1

Assessing Personal Feelings About HIV Prevention Education

◆ OVERVIEW

Students examine the importance of HIV prevention education in combating the AIDS epidemic, and brainstorm reasons why some teachers are concerned about providing this education. Then students complete handouts to identify personal feelings about teaching about HIV and AIDS education. In a subsequent discussion volunteers share *I Learned...* statements, which are open ended.

◆ OBJECTIVES

• Students analyze how personal feelings about HIV prevention education might affect their performance as teachers.

◆ MATERIALS

Handout: **Why Elementary/Middle School Teachers Might Choose** *Not* **to Teach About HIV and AIDS** (one for each student)

◆ ACTIVITIES

1. Begin class by writing HIV and AIDS on the chalkboard. Use the following dialogue to help frame an introduction to HIV prevention education. Using your own words, address all the important points presented in the dialogue.

    There is no good reason for anyone in this room who is not infected now to ever become infected with human immunodeficiency virus (HIV) or develop acquired immunodeficiency syndrome (AIDS). And there is no reason why any of the children in our schools should ever become infected with HIV or develop AIDS. Yet today's young people might become the next group to be hard:hit by HIV—the virus that causes AIDS. Why? A significant proportion of our young people engage in behaviors that can result in their becoming infected with HIV. *You*, as future teachers, can have a major impact on controlling the spread of HIV by helping our young people learn how to reduce and eliminate the risk of infection.

    By building and reinforcing self:esteem in our children, we can teach them that they are worth taking care of themselves. By developing their decision:making and refusal skills, we can give them the tools necessary to avoid risky behaviors. By giving them specific information about HIV infection and prevention, we can give them the facts they need to make informed choices.

    Yet some teachers are choosing not to teach about HIV infection and AIDS. In fact, some are *refusing* to teach about AIDS.

2. Have the students brainstorm reasons why kindergarten through eighth grade teachers might choose not to teach about HIV and AIDS. Record these reasons on the chalkboard. If their ideas do not include the following, guide students to include them.
    *   Kids have enough to worry about.
    *   It's not a problem in my town.
    *   Kids aren't interested in HIV.
    *   There's no room in my full schedule.
    *   I'm uncomfortable with death education.
    *   I'm uncomfortable with sex education.
    *   I lack knowledge about HIV and AIDS.
    *   This topic is not relevant to kids.

- This topic should be taught at home (not teacher's responsibility).
- I might be asked a question that I don't want to deal with.
- Parents and community might not be supportive.
- Since there is no cure for AIDS, I cannot offer hope.
- My school has no clear policy regarding what I can and cannot teach about AIDS.

Distribute the handout—**Why Elementary/Middle School Teachers Might Choose *Not* to Teach About HIV and AIDS**. Have students copy the list of reasons onto the handout.

3. Have students complete the handout by circling the number that best describes their feelings about each concern.

4. Have students analyze their responses to statements on the handout **Why Elementary/Middle School Teachers Might Choose *Not* to Teach About HIV and AIDS**. They should then write *I Learned...* statements about their responses. Ask volunteers to share any of the *I Learned...* statements that they feel comfortable sharing.

5. Reassure students that when people have a clear understanding of what HIV prevention education really involves, concern often gives way to confidence. Tell the students that after examining HIV and AIDS education in detail, you will return to this activity to discuss issues that continue to be of concern to them.

Why Elementary/Middle
School Teachers Might
Choose *Not* to Teach
About HIV and AIDS
handout

Why Elementary/Middle School Teachers Might Choose *Not* to Teach About HIV and AIDS

Directions: On the lines below, list reasons that teachers might give for deciding *not* to teach about HIV and AIDS. Then circle the number at the right of each reason to show how *you* might feel...as a kindergarten through third grade teacher and then as a fourth through eighth grade teacher.

1 = I would still teach about HIV and AIDS.

2 = This would cause me to be uncomfortable in teaching about HIV and AIDS.

3 = This would make me choose *not* to teach about HIV and AIDS.

	as a K-3 teacher	as a 4-8 teacher
_____	1 2 3	1 2 3
_____	1 2 3	1 2 3
_____	1 2 3	1 2 3
_____	1 2 3	1 2 3
_____	1 2 3	1 2 3
_____	1 2 3	1 2 3
_____	1 2 3	1 2 3
_____	1 2 3	1 2 3
_____	1 2 3	1 2 3
_____	1 2 3	1 2 3
_____	1 2 3	1 2 3
_____	1 2 3	1 2 3
_____	1 2 3	1 2 3
_____	1 2 3	1 2 3
_____	1 2 3	1 2 3

CHAPTER 2 *HIV Prevention Education: Scope and Sequence*

♦ **OVERVIEW**

Students examine the purpose of HIV prevention education, brainstorm appropriate content, and study the differences between HIV-specific and HIV-related content. Then students review the **Health Framework** transparency and explore how HIV-related content and HIV-specific content fit into a comprehensive school health education curriculum. Finally, students discuss considerations for an AIDS education program.

◇◇ Comprehensive school health education is "health education carried out in a school setting that is planned and carried out with the purpose of maintaining, reinforcing or enhancing the practices of children and youth that are conducive to their good health." It focuses on the entire continuum of health status and not merely on disease identification and prevention. The three interdependent components of comprehensive school health include:

Health Education (Instruction)
Community Health
Consumer Health
Environmental Health

Family Life
Growth and Development
Nutritional Health
Personal Health
Prevention and Control of Disease and Disorder
Safety and Accident Prevention
Substance Use and Abuse

Health Services
Health Appraisal-Medical Exam
Screenings
Teacher-Nurse Conference
Health Guidance
Communicable Disease Control
Emergency Care and Disaster Procedures

Healthful School Environment
Quality of School Site and Building
Gyms, Fields, Equipment
Lighting, Heating, Ventilation
School Food Services
Sanitation
Safety and Fire Protection
Mental-Emotional Tone
Health of School Personnel

◇◇Source: National Professional School Health Education Organization. Comprehensive school health education. In *Health Education,* 15(6): 4-8.

A comprehensive school health education curriculum requires not only school personnel and students but also parents and communities to plan, implement, and evaluate it.   ◇◇

◆ OBJECTIVES

- Students explain the function of HIV-specific and HIV-related content within an effective HIV prevention education program.
- Students describe how HIV prevention education fits into the elementary curriculum.
- Students describe how HIV prevention education fits into the concept of comprehensive school health education.

◆ MATERIALS

Transparency: **Purpose of HIV Prevention Education**
Transparency: **Health Framework**
Overlay A: **HIV-Related Content**
Overlay B: **HIV-Specific Content**
Resource: **Health Framework** (illustration of completed transparency)
Handout: **Sample Content Outline** (one for each student)
Handout: **Cultural Sensitivity for HIV Prevention Educators** (one for each student)

◆ ACTIVITIES

1. Provide an overview using the **Purpose of HIV Prevention Education** transparency.

   Explain that for children in early elementary school, students should learn to:
   - respond to questions directly and simply (limit answers to what is asked and to the developmental level of the child)
   - provide basic information to serve as a foundation for later HIV and AIDS information
   - eliminate unnecessary fears

   For children in upper elementary and middle school, students should learn to:
   - develop an understanding of the epidemiology of AIDS, HIV transmission, and the prevention of HIV infection
   - balance recognition of susceptibility to HIV infection with a sense of personal control in preventing infection

   Illustrate the importance of balancing feelings of susceptibility and control. Remind students that some people are so afraid of certain diseases that they refuse to participate in recommended screening procedures because they fear they might find they have the disease. For example, some women may fail to do monthly breast self-exams because they fear they might discover a lump. (*Note:* Example is for use by the college student, not those they teach.)

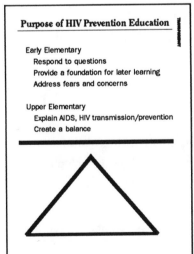

Purpose of HIV Prevention Education transparency

Illustrate on the transparency by writing CONTROL on one arm of the scale and SUSCEPTIBILITY on the other.

2. Write HIV-SPECIFIC on the board. Explain that HIV-specific content relates directly to characteristics of HIV infection and AIDS, to methods of transmission and prevention, and to other issues unique to HIV infection.

   Explain to students that classroom teachers have found that not all children have the basic information needed to help them understand the HIV-specific content. And not all children have the attitudes needed to adopt healthful behaviors. Illustrate this with the following examples:

   Ryane's teacher was puzzled by Ryane's difficulty in understanding the transmission of HIV, until the teacher realized that Ryane lacked the basic understanding that viruses are germs and that germs cause sickness.

   Jesse's teacher realized that before she could help Jesse adopt safe behaviors, she would have to help Jesse build self-esteem to the point where he liked himself enough to want to take care of himself.

   Write HIV-RELATED on the board. Explain that HIV-related information provides a foundation for learning HIV-specific information. It also encompasses material that contributes to a mature response to the AIDS crisis—such as decision-making skills, self-esteem, compassion for the ill, and refusal skills.

   Conclude that an effective HIV and AIDS curriculum reflects a combination of HIV-related and HIV-specific content. On the board, add the necessary notations to create the following formula:

   HIV-RELATED + HIV-SPECIFIC = HIV CURRICULUM CONTENT

3. Give the following examples of HIV-related content. Have students identify the concepts presented and how they relate to, but are not specific to, HIV infection.

   • In discussing *germs* with early elementary students, a teacher explains:
     Germs are living things that are so small we usually cannot see them except with a microscope. If you have ever seen moldy bread

or other food, that mold is a type of germ. There are many types of germs. Some grow in or on people and can make us sick. Our bodies have openings that are warm and wet—mouths, eyes, noses, and other places that we don't see because they are covered by our clothes.

Some germs live in warm, wet places. Some live in cool, dry places like the surface of our skin.

Germs can spread from one person to another person. The warm, wet places on our bodies have linings where certain germs can grow rapidly. If the germs in these places start growing (called an infection), they can make us sick.

- In a mental health lesson, children read and roleplay scenarios about peer pressure. They practice resisting peer pressure and brainstorm ways to avoid high-pressure situations.

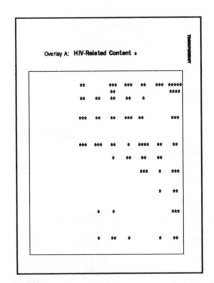

Health Framework
Transparency

4. Explain to students that as a district advisory committee decides how to organize curriculum content, they might examine how it fits into the ten traditional content areas of health education. Use the **Health Framework** transparency to explain or review these areas.

Adding Overlay A, **HIV-Related Content**, illustrate the placement of HIV-related content as it might appear in an existing comprehensive health education curriculum. (The **Sample Content Outline** shows what each star on the overlay represents. HIV-related content is preceded with an *R* on the handout.) Give the following examples:

Psychological Aspects of Personal Health
- why sick people need friends
- feelings associated with illness/death
- disease-related fears
- decision-making process
- psychological impact of illness in the family
- peer pressure
- setting life goals (lifestyle choices)

Personal Health
- recognizing uncomfortable touch
- positive health habits
- sense of responsibility for own health
- cleanliness
- variation in levels of wellness

Overlay A, **HIV-Related Content**

Growth and Development
- cells
- immune system parts and functions
- circulatory system parts and functions

Provide examples of HIV-related content from other categories, as appropriate.

5. Place Overlay B, **HIV-Specific Content,** on top of Overlay A, **HIV-Related Content**, and the **Health Framework** transparency. Explain that the overlay highlights the HIV-specific content.

Discuss the following questions:
- Does education about HIV and AIDS fit best in any single content area? (No. It builds on all categories.)
- If children were already receiving comprehensive health education, how much time would it take to teach HIV-specific content? (It would depend on the teaching methods selected, but generally, HIV-specific content could be covered in a partial lesson in lower grades. It might require two or three lessons in the upper elementary and middle school grades.)
- If only this HIV-specific content were taught and the school did *not* have a comprehensive health education curriculum, how would you rate the AIDS education program? (Weak. The children would be given a narrow view of AIDS and HIV without a broader context that can enhance understanding.)
- Is HIV prevention education synonymous with sex education? (No. The Family Life category [see **Health Framework**] provides HIV-related content, and most of this material is a prerequisite for HIV prevention education. For example, teach elementary school children the appropriate names for genitalia, teach late elementary school children the meaning of the term *sexual intercourse*.)

Conclude that HIV prevention education should be presented in the context of comprehensive school health education.

Point out to students that when HIV and AIDS are presented in the context of other health issues rather than as a separate "crisis" topic, the subject appears less overwhelming and alarming to children, parents, and teachers. Within a comprehensive school health education curriculum, developmentally appropriate material is presented

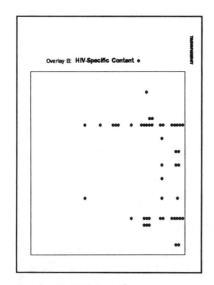

Overlay B, **HIV-Specific Content**

sequentially so that earlier content has laid a foundation for understanding HIV-specific information. Therefore, these concepts will not be entirely new.

6. Explain that before specific teaching methods are selected for a curriculum, a number of factors might provide direction when selecting appropriate teaching strategies. For example:

   • In addition to adding HIV content (related and specific) to a comprehensive school health education curriculum, *HIV prevention education can be integrated* into several areas of the total curriculum. Art, math, science, and social studies provide such opportunities. HIV infection has many social and political ramifications—thus, it is a topic that will correlate with a variety of classroom subjects. Incorporating HIV material into the context of other issues helps reinforce concepts provided in health education lessons.

   Distribute copies of the **Sample Content Outline.** Ask students to describe other content areas in the elementary curriculum where HIV prevention education could be integrated.

   • *Teachable moments* are effective in teaching young children what they need to know when they are most interested. A teachable moment occurs when a child's question or comment provides the teacher with an opportunity to add information, or clarify and correct misinformation.

   • *The regular classroom teacher can best orchestrate HIV prevention education in the elementary school classroom.* Information about HIV infection must be presented on many occasions and in many formats by sources credible to young children. The classroom teacher, who is constantly accessible, well-versed in teaching methods, aware of individual childrens' abilities, and trusted as a source of reliable information, serves as the ideal person to select the most appropriate methods to convey this critical information.

   • *No one curriculum is best.* HIV and AIDS curricula must meet the needs of the children and respond to the values and concerns of the community.

   • *New teaching skills are not required.* HIV prevention education should be taught in many different ways, through as many different vehicles as possible, but new teaching methods are not required. Teachers who use the same three or four teaching methods, however, may want to add to their repertoire, because some methods may be more appropriate than others.

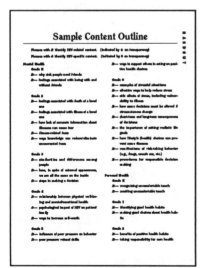

Sample Content Outline
handout

- *Coeducational classes* are important to foster both male and female responsibility for preventing HIV infection.
- *Language* must be precise. Some terms such as *body fluids, casual contact, PLWA* (Person Living with AIDS), and *sex industry worker* (prostitute) can interfere with learning if children don't know what the words mean. For example, the statement "One way to avoid HIV is to abstain from sexual intercourse" uses appropriate and correct terms, but children who do not yet know the meaning of the terms will not understand the statement. Also, children who have not been taught that AIDS is a preventable disease may feel undue anxiety if they are told that "people are dying from AIDS." They might conclude that parent/teacher "aides" in their schools are dying or killing people. Similarly, how secure will children feel when their teacher leaves the classroom after an announcement which asks, "Will all teachers with aides come to the office?"

Vulgar and inappropriate language may be used when children do not know proper terms. A suggested approach is for the teacher to say to the child, "In this class, we use the term _____." When everyone learns proper terms, it will become easier to discuss children's concerns.

- *AIDS* is the term that designates the disease acquired immunodeficiency syndrome. Scientists have come to understand that HIV infection predates AIDS by months or years. The term *HIV infection* has become more commonly used. In the elementary school, the term *AIDS* may be used until the AIDS virus is introduced as HIV and the stages of infection are identified in the lessons.
- Teachers need to be sensitive to signs of *resentment* in young people, who naturally dislike being told how to behave (specifically, to abstain from sex and intravenous drug use). Individuals like to make their own behavior choices. The false feeling of immortality common to many young people makes them especially vulnerable to feelings of resentment.
- *Abstinence* from sex and from intravenous drug use is to be promoted. If alternate means of protection are presented, these alternatives are not to be offered as equal choices to abstinence, but as second choices that are less preferable and less reliable. This position regarding abstinence takes into consideration the physical and emotional maturity of children and the moral standards of most communities.
- Some states have laws requiring *notification of parents* prior to instruction about sexually transmitted disease. It is *essential* to pro-

vide parents with an opportunity to review instructional materials and to comply with any parental request that you excuse a child from HIV prevention education. Parental support is important.

- *Parent-child communication can be encouraged* by giving children specific assignments or activities to do with their parents. However, some parents may not want to discuss HIV and AIDS with their children (because they feel uncomfortable or because they feel they do not have adequate information). Teachers need to reassure the children that it is all right if their parents choose not to discuss HIV and AIDS with them.

- Children need to learn that *protecting oneself is normal behavior*. Through comprehensive health education, children learn to recognize that it is normal and healthy to take care of oneself and others.

- *Teachers must be sensitive* to the values and practices of varying cultures when addressing all subjects. It is particularly important when addressing HIV and AIDS. Distribute copies of the **Cultural Sensitivity for HIV Prevention Educators** handout. Tell students this information can increase their awareness of cultural issues around HIV prevention education.

- Teachers serve an important role in recognizing *children who have special concerns* or who need more detailed information because of their high-risk behavior, environment, attitudes, or beliefs. Children who express concern about loved ones or who seem confused about HIV information should also receive additional attention. Teachers should follow school policy in referring children to local resources for assistance or support.

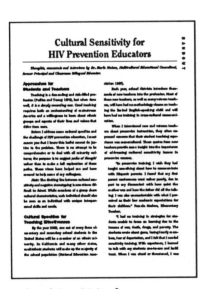

Cultural Sensitivity for HIV Prevention Educators handout

Purpose of HIV Prevention Education

Early Elementary

    Respond to questions

    Provide a foundation for later learning

    Address fears and concerns

Upper Elementary

    Explain AIDS, HIV transmission/prevention

    Create a balance

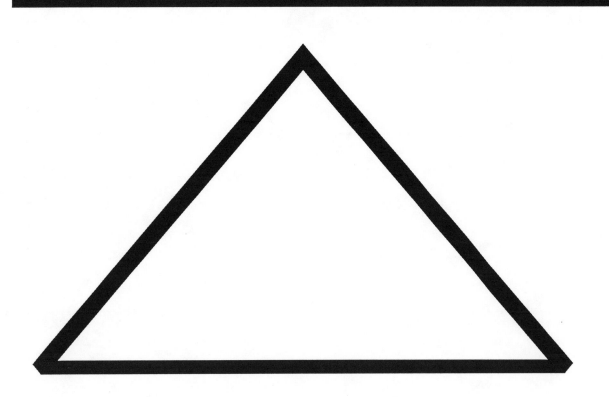

Health Framework

	K	1	2	3	4	5	6
Mental Health							
Personal Health							
Disease							
Nutrition							
Drugs							
Family Life							
Growth and Development							
Safety and First Aid							
Community/ Environmental Health							
Consumer Health							

Overlay A: **HIV-Related Content** ★

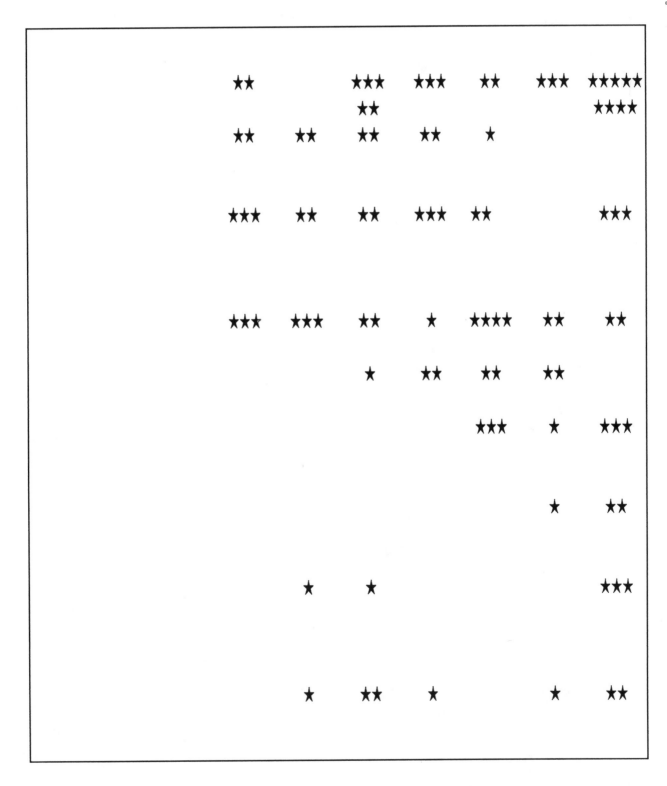

Overlay B: **HIV-Specific Content** ●

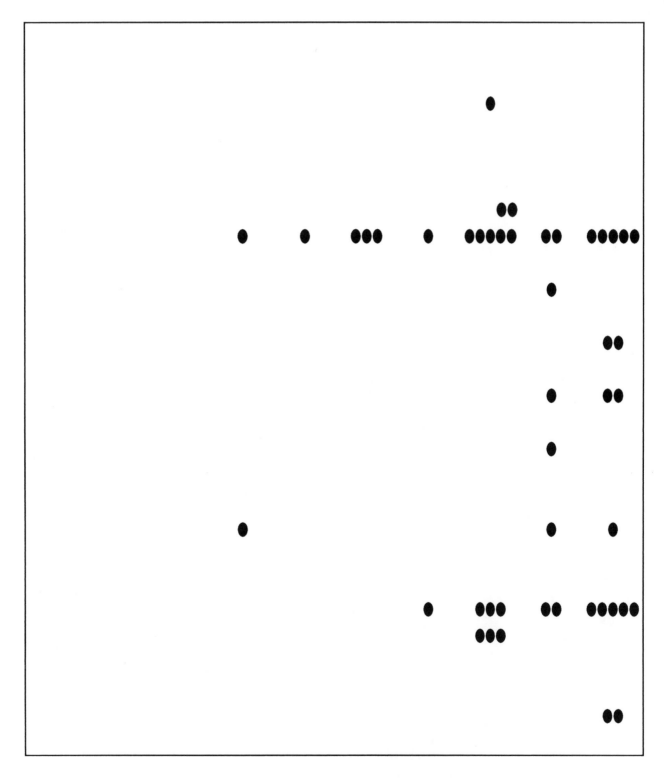

Health Framework

Overlay A: **HIV-Related Content** ★
Overlay B: **HIV-Specific Content** ●

	K	1	2	3	4	5	6
Mental Health	★★		★★★ ★★	★★★	★★ ●	★★★	★★★★★ ★★★★
Personal Health	★★	★★	★★	★★	★		
Disease	★★★ ●	★★ ●	★★ ●●●	★★★ ●	★★ ●● ●●●●●	●●	★★★ ●●●●●
Nutrition						●	
Drugs	★★★	★★★	★★	★	★★★★	★★	★★ ●●
Family Life			★	★★	★★	★★ ●	●●
Growth and Development					★★★	★ ●	★★★
Safety and First Aid	●					★ ●	★★ ●
Community/ Environmental Health		★	★	●	●●● ●●●	●●	★★★ ●●●●●
Consumer Health		★	★★	★		★	★★ ●●

Sample Content Outline

Phrases with **R** identify HIV-related content. (indicated by ★ on transparency)

Phrases with **S** identify HIV-specific content. (indicated by ◑ on transparency)

Mental Health

Grade K

R— why sick people need friends

R— feelings associated with being with and without friends

Grade 2

R— feelings associated with death of a loved one

R— feelings associated with illness of a loved one

R— how lack of accurate information about illnesses can cause fear

R— disease-related fears

R— ways knowledge can reduce/eliminate unwarranted fears

Grade 3

R— similarities and differences among people

R— how, in spite of external appearances, we are all the same on the inside

R— steps in making a decision

Grade 4

R— relationship between physical well-being and mental/emotional health

S— psychological impact of HIV on patient/ family

R— ways to increase self-worth

Grade 5

R— influence of peer pressure on behavior

R— peer pressure refusal skills

R— ways to support others in acting on positive health choices

Grade 6

R— examples of stressful situations

R— effective ways to help reduce stress

R— side effects of stress, including vulnerability to illness

R— how some decisions must be altered if circumstances change

R— short-term and long-term consequences of decisions

R— the importance of setting realistic life goals

R— how lifestyle (health) choices can prevent some diseases

R— ramifications of risk-taking behavior (e.g., drugs, unsafe sex, etc.)

R— procedures for responsible decision making

Personal Health

Grade K

R— recognizing uncomfortable touch

R— avoiding uncomfortable touch

Grade 1

R— identifying good health habits

R— making good choices about health habits

Grade 2

R— benefits of positive health habits

R— taking responsibility for own health

Grade 3

R— physical, mental, social implications of cleanliness

R— good health habits (such as exercise, relaxation, sleep, diet)

Grade 4

R— variation in levels of wellness

Disease Prevention and Control

Grade K

R— defining germs

R— ways to avoid germs

S— the nature of germs

R— the need for cleanliness

Grade 1

S— ways to break the communicable disease cycle

R— fears about casual transmission of many diseases

R— diseases that are communicable and those that are not

Grade 2

R— sound health habits that can help prevent disease

R— ways senses "listen to" our bodies to monitor health

S— AIDS as a disease that is causing adults to get very sick

S— the name of the germ that causes AIDS (HIV)

S— that HIV infection is not common among children

Grade 3

R— the difference between communicable disease and chronic degenerative disease

R— bacteria and viruses as specific kinds of germs

R— how disease can be categorized by cause (virus, bacteria)

S— casual contact not being a way that HIV is spread

Grade 4

R— certain viruses that cause disease among people

R— viruses too small to be visualized except with powerful microscopes

R— transmission of viruses

S— the small number of doctors, nurses, and other medical personnel who have been infected when they were directly exposed to HIV-infected blood

S— the virus that causes AIDS

S— the ability of HIV to weaken an infected person's immune system

S— symptoms that are indicators that disease is present

S— how it sometimes takes several years after becoming infected with HIV before symptoms appear

S— the symptoms of HIV infection and AIDS

S— HIV not transmitted in the same ways as some other more familiar viruses, e.g., flu viruses and measles viruses that are transmitted through the air

Grade 5

S— how HIV-infected people can infect other people—even though they do not look or feel sick

S— why people infected with HIV get diseases that do not normally affect people with healthy immune systems

Grade 6

R— the serious consequences of infections that are transmittable through contact with blood

S— why so many HIV-infected people who developed AIDS lived only a few years after being diagnosed

R— how lifestyle choices can be health risks

S— ways to prevent the spread of HIV include saying no to sex and drugs

R— social and cultural forces in the development of responsible health behavior (including sexual behavior)

R— ways to prevent sexually transmitted diseases (STDs)

S— abstinence as the most effective way to prevent sexual transmission of HIV and STDs

R— choosing mature and responsible sexual behavior

Nutrition

Grade 5

S— opportunistic diseases that cause diarrhea in patients with HIV infection

S: wasting syndrome as a manifestation of AIDS

Drugs

Grade K

R— how the use of unknown substances can be hazardous

R— appropriate use of medicines

R— the importance of avoiding the use of unknown or hazardous substances

Grade 1

R— defining abuse

R— substances that people abuse

R— how to make decisions about helpful and harmful drugs

Grade 2

R— difference between drug use, drug misuse, drug abuse

R— dangers of abuse of potentially harmful substances

Grade 3

R— pleasurable activities to be used in unstructured time

Grade 5

R— effect of drugs on body systems

S— role of IV drugs and needles/syringes in the transmission of HIV

R— refusal skills

R— the roles of individuals in preventing the abuse of substances

Grade 6

R— hazards associated with use of drugs, alcohol, tobacco

S— how HIV can be transmitted by sharing IV drug paraphernalia

S— physical, mental, social effects of drug use (including HIV infection)

S— IV drug use as high-risk behavior (due to HIV transmission)

Family Life

Grade 2

R— ways each family member depends on other family members

Grade 3

R— unique social and physical characteristics of boys and girls

R— ways of dealing with feelings associated with serious illness, death, grief

Grade 4

R— growth spurt that occurs during adolescence

R— supportive attitudes toward family members

Grade 5

R— function of the reproductive system

R— role of abstinence in the prevention of sexually transmitted diseases (STDs)

S— sexual intercourse

Grade 6

R— transmission of HIV from mother to infant before or during birth

S— how condoms can keep HIV from being passed

Growth and Development

Grade 4

R— ways growth and development occur at the level of the cell

R— structure of the immune system

R— how the immune system helps the body fight off disease

Grade 5

R— ways the immune system functions (including how antibodies and white blood cells such as macrophages do their jobs)

S— how HIV affects the immune system

Grade 6

R— role of blood in transporting nutrients, waste products, hormones, and drugs

R— structure and function of the circulatory system

S— how HIV is transmitted through blood

Safety and First Aid

Grade K

R— what to do in emergencies where bleeding occurs

Grade 5

R— importance of taking responsibility for safety of self and others

S— importance of preventing infection with HIV to protect self and others

Grade 6

R— importance of following first aid measures for bleeding and shock

Community Health

Grade 1

R— school health personnel and their services

Grade 2

R— roles of health helpers in the community

Grade 3

S— lack of vaccine to prevent HIV infection and lack of a cure for HIV infection or AIDS

Grade 4

S— how scientists all over the world are working to find a way to stop people from becoming infected with HIV and to cure those who are infected

S— how HIV infection is occurring worldwide (in every state in U.S. and in most other countries of the world)

S— occurrence of HIV infection in cities, suburbs, small towns, and urban areas

S— the likelihood of teenagers becoming infected with HIV (although most infected people are adults)

S— how HIV affects females as well as males

S— how HIV affects people of every race

Grade 5

S— estimated number of people in the U.S. who are infected with HIV

S— HIV infection as a community health problem

Grade 6

R— role of community health agencies in protecting and promoting the health and safety of community members

S— local health facilities that provide assistance to HIV-infected people

S— services available for AIDS- related needs

R— importance of individual participation in community health activities

R— ways that young people can help meet community health needs

S— how HIV cannot be contracted by donating blood

S— the impact of HIV and AIDS on a community

S— medical, technical, and other careers that provide opportunities to join the fight against AIDS

Consumer Health

Grade 1

R— services provided by health care workers

Grade 2

R— ways to accept responsibility for one's own health

R— ways the media influences decisions

Grade 3

R— sources of health information

Grade 5

R— situations in which activities that promote well-being are likely to occur

Grade 6

R— reliability and credibility of media sources for HIV information

S— claims for "miracle cures" for HIV infection

S— establishment of regulations to prevent the transmission of HIV through blood transfusions

R— costs of preventative versus therapeutic health care

Cultural Sensitivity for HIV Prevention Educators

*Thoughts, comments and interviews by **Dr. Maria Natera**, Multicultural Educational Consultant, former Principal and Classroom Bilingual Educator.*

Approaches for Students and Teachers

Teaching is a demanding and risk-filled profession (Pullias and Young 1976), but when done well, *it is a deeply rewarding one.* Good teaching requires both an understanding of mainstream America and a willingness to learn about ethnic groups and aspects of their lives and values that differ from ours.

Before I address some cultural specifics and the challenge of HIV prevention education, I must assure you that I know this leaflet cannot do justice to the problem. There is no attempt to be comprehensive or to deal with all minority cultures; the purpose is to suggest *paths of thought* rather than to make a full exploration of those paths. These views have helped me and have seemed to help some of my colleagues.

Note: The dividing line between cultural sensitivity and negative stereotyping is sometimes difficult to detect. While members of a group share cultural characteristics, each individual should also be seen as an individual with unique interpersonal skills and needs.

Cultural Specifics for Teaching Effectiveness

By the year 2000, one out of every three elementary and secondary school students in the United States will be a member of an ethnic minority. In California and many other states, multiethnic students will make up the majority of the school population (National Education Association 1987).

Each year, school districts introduce thousands of new teachers into the profession. Most of these new teachers, as well as many veteran teachers, will have had no methodology classes on teaching the limited English-speaking child and will have had no training in cross-cultural communication.

When I interviewed new and veteran teachers about preservice instruction, they often expressed concern that their student teaching experience was monocultural. These quotes from new teachers provide some insight into the importance of addressing cultural sensitivity issues in preservice courses.

"In preservice training, I wish they had taught something about how to communicate with Hispanic parents. I found that my first parent conferences went rather poorly, due in part to my discomfort with how quiet the mother was and how the father did all the talking. I was also uncomfortable with what I perceived as their low academic expectations for their children." Pamela Madera, Elementary Teacher.

"I had no training in strategies for students unable to focus on learning due to the trauma of war, death, drugs, and poverty. The students wrote about guns, losing family members, fear of deportation, and I felt that I needed sensitivity training. With experience, I learned to talk with my students one-to-one and build trust. When I was afraid or threatened, I was quite distant from my students and with their parents." Ellen Gee, High School Teacher.

"Students know when I am uncomfortable with them—how sometimes I don't understand them, their parents or their apathy or poverty. Before I can teach them, I must get to know them." Deb Clay, Middle School Teacher.

"In preservice training, I didn't learn to work with language and cultural differences. Fortunately, my district has a program for new teachers. However, I have three friends in another district who were dynamic just a year ago in graduate school, but are planning to leave the profession at the end of the year, due to the difficult assignments, the unrealistic preservice program, and the lack of a supportive program at their schools." Kenneth Williams, Elementary Teacher.

Future teachers need help in comprehending the complexities of their first assignments, including a cultural exploration of who their students are and why they act the way they do. The United States is a multicultural community.

According to Edward T. Hall in *Beyond Culture* (1981), the study of cultures and the consideration of ethnicities is especially important for Americans, because they are generally intolerant of differences and have a tendency to consider something different as inferior. U.S. schools use competition as a primary method for motivating students and stress the importance of the individual. These values are part of American culture and are not shared by all cultures.

Many of our values may be unconscious, which can increase the difficulty of intercultural communication. Therefore, cross-cultural learning in the schools becomes a necessity. Cultural sensitivity means more than education, teaching or training. In multiethnic classrooms, cultural sensitivity means that the **how** of communication is at least as important as the **what**.

Seven Capacities for Cultural Sensitivity

I am convinced that teachers inevitably teach lessons based on their own beliefs and values. Hence, a commitment to becoming culturally sensitive is an essential ingredient in your success as a teacher. As you consider the following *capacities,* do some personal introspection. Ask yourself, "Which capacities are currently my personal qualities? Which ones might need further development? How might I, as a future teacher, develop a greater level of cultural sensitivity?"

1. *The capacity to communicate respect*: to transmit, verbally and nonverbally, positive regard, encouragement, and sincere interest.
2. *The capacity to personalize knowledge and perceptions*: to recognize the influence of one's own values, perceptions, opinions, and knowledge of human interaction, and to regard such as relative, rather than absolute.
3. *The capacity to display empathy*: to try to understand others from their point of view, to attempt to put oneself into others' life space and to feel as they do about the matter under consideration.
4. *The capacity to be nonjudgmental*: to avoid value-laden, evaluative statements, which may cause internal conflicts, and to listen in such a way that others (students, colleagues, or friends) can fully share and explain themselves.
5. *The capacity for role flexibility*: to be able to get a task accomplished in a manner and time frame appropriate to the learner, and to be flexible in the process for getting assignments done, particularly with reference to participation and group activities.
6. *The capacity to demonstrate reciprocal concern*: to take turns talking, share the responsibility for interaction, and in group work, promote circular communication. Refining

listening skills reinforces the capacity to demonstrate reciprocal concern.

7. ***The capacity to tolerate ambiguity***: to be able to cope with cultural differences, to accept a degree of frustration, and to deal with ever-changing circumstances and people.

(Adapted from the Canadian International Development Agency model as described in *Managing Cultural Differences*, Harris and Moran 1979.)

These capacities overlap and interrelate. Consider the variety of capacities addressed in the following examples:

- Teachers have many ways of showing trust and respect to students. Teachers communicate respect and trust in the way they respond to questions, the privileges they grant, and the way they express discontent. They have a responsibility to communicate their respect for the variety of cultures represented in their classrooms.

- Different cultures have different values, beliefs, and characteristics. Teachers need to understand the cultural backgrounds of their students. They should be aware of and sensitive to religious beliefs and customs and considerate of home situations.

Many factors in our society have contributed to a reduction in the amount of time parents spend with their children. Single parents may not be able to devote much time to assist children with homework. Parents with limited English ability may not be able to assist their children with certain assignments. Teachers need to consider these factors when planning lessons and making assignments.

- When addressing issues related to disease, it is important to remember that different cultures have different belief systems regarding disease and illness. It may be necessary to assume the learner role and allow students to share their belief systems. This enlightenment will enable the teacher to adapt lessons to allow for multicultural beliefs, thus promoting a better understanding of disease.

- To provide models for effective group interaction, teachers must permit themselves to assume the learner role in order to hear and develop an understanding of the attitudes, beliefs, and values of their students that are dictated by cultural factors. Each student should be encouraged to work as a member of the group to achieve certain goals. By being alert and sensitive, teachers can provide opportunities for students to express themselves and to clarify their feelings.

"Culture teaches us what to value, and what to fear, which behavior signals to watch for in others, and which to send, which words to use and which to avoid" (Harris and Moran 1979). It is important to recognize the attitudes we hold and assumptions we make about other groups. These assumptions usually are unconscious. The importance of our behavior is apparent in the saying: "Your actions speak so loudly, I can hardly hear what you say." We must see ourselves as others see us before we can seek an objective view of our students.

HIV Issues and Minority Populations

"AIDS is disproportionately affecting People of Color, particularly in the African-American and Hispanic communities" (Gerald 1988). The County of Los Angeles Commission on Human Relations held a hearing on AIDS and the minority populations in winter 1988. According to Carol Chang,

Human Relations Commissioner, some commonalties surfaced as representatives from the African-American, Latino, Native American, Asian, and Pacific Islander communities testified.

The most alarming common thread in the testimony was the difficulty these communities have in acknowledging the problem of HIV. This is due in part to cultural stigmas and lack of knowledge. Latino health workers reported that it is very difficult for some Latinos to accept ideas that contradict moral beliefs. For example, Latino women cannot bring themselves to suggest the use of condoms because they are not supposed to know about such things as sex, homosexuality, and substance abuse.

These minority groups also have difficulty acknowledging homosexuality (Chang 1989). The invisibility of homosexuals, because many do not self-identify as gay or bisexual even though they may engage in sex with other males, complicates the issue.

Drug usage is a concern among these groups, particularly as it relates to HIV. Pacific Islanders (Samoans) report a high level of intravenous drug usage. Thirty-six percent of the African-American and Latino cases of AIDS occur among intravenous drug users, compared to only 6 percent among whites (Gerald 1988). Native American groups with high numbers of substance abusers report a need to have the mainstream culture help strengthen their social culture, not to destroy it, as they learn about the dangers of HIV (National Education Association 1987).

The commission also found that in minority communities medical resources are often inadequate, and community members feel isolated and generally do not have health insurance. "The AIDS health crisis exacerbates the underlying poor health and poor socioeconomic conditions among America's racial and ethnic minorities" (Gerald 1988).

Clearly, culturally sensitive education about HIV and AIDS must be directed at all members of our population if we are to effectively stop the spread of this terrible disease. It is imperative that HIV and AIDS information and education be available to minorities by early adolescence. For HIV prevention messages to effectively reach the minority populations, general education programs must be reinforced by culturally sensitive teaching strategies.

References

California State Department of Education. 1987. *California beginning teacher assessment and support project*. Sacramento, CA.

Chang, C. 1989. Interview. Testimony by representatives of minority communities to the L.A. County Commission on Human Relations. Los Angeles, CA.

Gerald, G. R. 1988. Minority populations: AIDS risks and prevention. In *The AIDS challenge*, ed. Quackenbush, M., M. Nelson and K. Clark. Santa Cruz, CA: Network Publications, a division of ETR Associates.

Hall, E. T. 1981. *Beyond culture*. Garden City, NY: Anchor Books.

Harris, P. and R. T. Moran. 1979. *Managing cultural differences*. Houston: Gulf Publishing Company.

National Education Association (NEA). 1987. Executive Committee Study Group Reports on Ethnic Minority. *And justice for all*. Washington, DC.

Pullias, E. V. and J. D. Young. 1976. *A teacher is many things*. London, IN: Indiana University Press.

Responding to Children's Questions

CHAPTER 3

◆ OVERVIEW

Students brainstorm the meaning behind children's questions and identify ways to respond to an unexpected question. Criteria for assessing the situation and examples of responses that do not foster continued communication are examined. Groups practice appropriate responses to questions and discuss the importance of follow-up.

◆ OBJECTIVES

- Students compose an appropriate response to a child's question about HIV or AIDS.
- Students describe guidelines for formulating an appropriate response to a child's question.

◆ MATERIALS

Transparency: **Question**
Overlay A: **Assess**
Resource: ***Real* Question** (illustration of completed transparency)

◆ ACTIVITIES

1. Explain that when responding to HIV-related questions, the classroom teacher needs:
   - a strong knowledge base of HIV content, which can be provided through preservice inservice training
   - a clear understanding of child development (a major component of teacher-training programs nationwide)
   - an approach that allows children to feel at ease in expressing their concerns and questions

   Teachers who feel ill-prepared in any of these three areas should notify their supervisors and seek additional training. No teacher should be forced to teach about HIV and AIDS without proper training. Some teachers might find team teaching a more comfortable situation for their first experiences.

2. In responding to any question, teachers must look for the *meaning* behind the words. For example, if four children ask, "What is the difference between boys and girls?" each child might mean something different. Quackenbush and Villarreal (1988) have identified possible motivations behind children's questions. These motivations are discussed in the following insert.

◇◇ **The Meaning of Children's Questions**
Some AIDS-related questions that arise with young children are presented below.

I. **Information-seeking and general curiosity**
Something stimulates the child's curiosity and there is a natural interest in finding out more. Questions of this nature may resemble: What is AIDS? How come gay men get AIDS? Why does God let babies die?

II. Anxiety for one's own welfare

Children wonder if they could get AIDS or if they will die. Questions falling in this category may include: Are people with AIDS bad? How do people get AIDS? What kind of people get AIDS?

III. Anxiety for the welfare of parents, siblings, other family members, and friends

Family is one of the most important aspects of a child's life. Discussion may prompt a concern for the well-being of friends and family. Some questions exhibiting these concerns may include: Will my mother get AIDS? Do all grown-ups know how not to get AIDS?

IV. Solution seeking

As children get to be about seven or eight, they begin to try to develop solutions to problems. Questions that may be part of the solution process will resemble: Could a very good doctor help someone with AIDS be healthy? Can we give someone with AIDS new blood to help them be better?

V. Seeking reactions from adults

Sometimes children enjoy baffling grown-ups with difficult or embarrassing questions. Sometimes they will ask such questions to examine how grown-ups react to subjects that are hard to talk about. Questions in this category should be addressed in a matter-of-fact and honest manner. This will cause children to lose interest in the game.

VI. Special psychological needs

Should a child become unusually anxious, AIDS may have become the focus of anxiety in his or her life. Such a child may repeatedly ask similar or identical questions, never seeming satisfied with the answer or never fully absorbing the information. If such questions persist over several weeks, a consultation with a child counselor may be called for.   ◇◇

◇◇Source: Quackenbush, M. and S. Villarreal. *"Does AIDS Hurt?"* Santa Cruz, Calif.: ETR Associates.

Have students brainstorm what the real meaning might be if a child asks, "How do people get AIDS?" For example, the child could be curious, worried about having AIDS, or worried about friends or family. The child also could be seeking solutions to the AIDS problem, trying to shock the teacher, measuring the teachers askability, or displaying concern that masks underlying psychological needs.

Emphasize that questions should be clarified, because the students need to learn to respond not to the words but to the real meaning behind them. Illustrate this with the following example:

When T.J. asked his teacher, "What is a homosexual?" Mrs. Kemp explored with T.J. the information he already had in order to learn why he was asking the question. She began by asking T.J. what he knew about homosexuals. T.J. said he had heard that homosexuals get AIDS and that homosexuals are people who love people of their same sex. T.J. was in the very normal stage of development at which he preferred to be with members of his same sex. He also loved his father. He was concerned that he was at risk because he loved his father and male friends. T.J. didn't need a detailed description of a homosexual lifestyle—he needed to be reassured that he is normal and not at risk.

The following are questions that children may ask. Have students discuss the meaning behind these questions. The questions and notes about the meanings are adapted from *"Does AIDS Hurt?"* (Quackenbush and Villareal, 1988.)

- Do people get AIDS from being bad?
  No. Some people get AIDS because the AIDS virus entered into their bodies somehow. People get AIDS from having sex with someone who has the disease. But sex isn't bad and neither are people who have sex.
  Some people get AIDS from using drugs and sharing needles with someone who has the AIDS germ. The people who do this are not bad, but using drugs is very dangerous.
  Note: *This question...may express a child's anxiety about his or her own "goodness" or "badness." Answers should be very reassuring.*
- What happens to children with AIDS?
  Children with AIDS are a lot like other children with serious diseases. They are often quite sick. They see doctors who help take care of them. Sometimes they have to stay in a hospital for awhile. When they feel better, they can go home again.
  Sometimes children with AIDS are so sick that the doctors can't make them better, and they die.
  Maybe you have heard about things that happen to children with AIDS. I wonder if you can tell me what you know.
  Note: *This is usually a question stemming from a child's anxiety about the terrible things that can happen to children in general. Many children have heard news stories about ostracism, neglect, or*

abandonment of children with AIDS. Answers to this question should seek to lower anxiety and avoid frightening or explicit detail.

3. Show the **Question** transparency and review the first step in responding to a question, which is to find out the real question that the child is asking. Write REAL to the left of the word *Question* on the transparency. (For an example of completed transparency, see the ***Real* Question** resource.)

    Using the transparency, explain that in most situations teachers will have anticipated questions and are prepared to respond. Write PREPARED in the upper left box on the transparency. However, some questions will come as a surprise. Write SURPRISED in the upper right box on the transparency. For difficult questions, a teacher should acknowledge the question and ask for more time to prepare an answer. Write ASK FOR MORE TIME on the transparency, as illustrated on the ***Real* Question** resource.

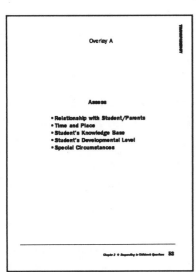

Question transparency

    Ask students for ways they might ask for more time.

    Ask students to suggest other examples.

4. Explain that once prepared, teachers should *assess the situation* to determine an appropriate response. Add Overlay A, **Assess**, to the transparency to provide content for "The Situation" box.

    "Does AIDS Hurt?" offers the following points to consider when preparing an appropriate response:

    1. Your relationship with the child.
    2. The particular circumstances at hand.
    3. Your own sense of preparedness.
    4. Your previous discussions with the child on this or related topics.
    5. The child's age and developmental level.
    6. Any special history pertinent to the circumstances.
    7. What is the real meaning behind the questions?

    Review these considerations with your students. Remind them that a child's age is merely a guide to be used in determining his or her level of sophistication.

Overlay A, **Assess**

Explain that by assessing the situation teachers can find appropriate answers that are sensitive to the concerns of parents and community. Point out that many parents who oppose HIV education are afraid their children will be given too much, too soon. Many parents are concerned that in answering questions of young children, teachers might frighten or upset them with talk of sex, disease, and death. Teachers who are sensitive to a child's developmental level realize that children generally are unable to comprehend death and reproduction until late in their elementary school years. Thus, describing AIDS as a disease that is making lots of people die is inappropriate for young children. Providing detailed explanations of sexual intercourse and intravenous drug use also is inappropriate in early elementary grades.

5.   Tell students that all responses to questions should meet two criteria:
  •   *Answers should be simple.* (Write SIMPLE after "#1" in the "Screen Your Response" box on the transparency.) Illustrate this point by sharing the example of Taralyn, a girl from Taiwan, who asked her adoptive American mother, "Where did I come from?" Taralyn's mom had prepared herself for the day she would answer this question for her daughter. Taralyn patiently listened as her mom explained reproduction in detail and then said, "Mom, I only wanted to know if I came from America or Taipei."
  •   *Answers should encourage continued conversation with grown-ups at home and school.* (Write ENCOURAGE CONVERSATION WITH PARENTS/SCHOOL after "#2" on the transparency.) Ask students to think of examples of answers that would *not* encourage continued conversation. For example:
    • When you get older, I'll tell you.
    • It's nothing you need be concerned about.
    • That's really not your business.
    • I didn't understand it when I was your age and I turned out okay.
    • You know.
    • Those are bad words, and I don't ever want you to say them.
    • Just wait. You'll find out when you need to know.

6.   Refer to the "Response" box on the transparency. Ask your students to think about how teachers should answer a kindergarten student's question, "How do people get AIDS?"

Recognizing that these same words can be asking different things, the teacher must first identify the real question by asking, "Are you worried that you might get AIDS?" or "Have you heard of some ways that the AIDS germ is spread?"

Once the child provides an answer, the teacher can correct misinformation and reassure the child that HIV and AIDS are not easily spread and are not common in children. The teacher should also encourage the child to continue sharing his or her concerns with grown-ups at home or school.

If the question seems to be based on curiosity, the teacher needs to keep in mind that students in early elementary grades are not developmentally ready for detailed information about sexual intercourse or intravenous drug use. The teacher might answer by saying:

Grown-ups understand exactly what germ causes AIDS and how it spreads. They know how to protect themselves. But it's hard for me to explain in words. Let's do this. We will learn about HIV and AIDS little by little. As you understand one idea, we will use that idea like a step that will get us to the next idea. Soon you will know exactly how to protect yourself and others from HIV and AIDS. Okay? Let's start by being sure that you know that HIV is not common in children. AIDS is a disease that mostly grown-ups get. It is caused by a virus that lives inside, not outside, the body of a person with AIDS. Let's first learn about ways germs spread and what you can do to stop the spread of germs.

7. Ask students what response would be appropriate if the teacher determines that a child's questions cannot be answered because school policy prohibits discussion of certain topics, such as sexual intercourse. Explain to students that the sensitivity of HIV and AIDS education evokes the establishment of policies by school systems that may influence the teacher's ability to respond to children's questions. When experiencing a conflict with the policies, the teacher should be truthful and respond by telling children that school rules prohibit him or her from discussing that topic in school. Teachers may want to share the child's concern with the parents. Have students discuss their reaction to that response.

Suggest that an alternative response might be to explain to the child that most parents want to share certain situations with their children—such as walking for the first time, losing the first tooth, learning how babies are made, and preparing for the first date. For this reason, when children indicate they are ready to learn about sex, schools refer questions back to parents.

Suggest that as follow-up, the teacher might offer to help the child initiate the discussion at home. The teacher should alert parents to a child's interest and make resources available. Stress that teacher follow-up in this situation is essential to ensure that the child's questions do not go unanswered.

Write FOLLOW-UP in the remaining box on the transparency.

8. As time allows, have students brainstorm other possible questions from children. They can practice responding in small groups.

9. Conclude that following the guidelines just outlined can help teachers feel confident in responding to children's questions. Ask for volunteers to summarize these guidelines in their own words. (This could also be a written assignment.)

Question

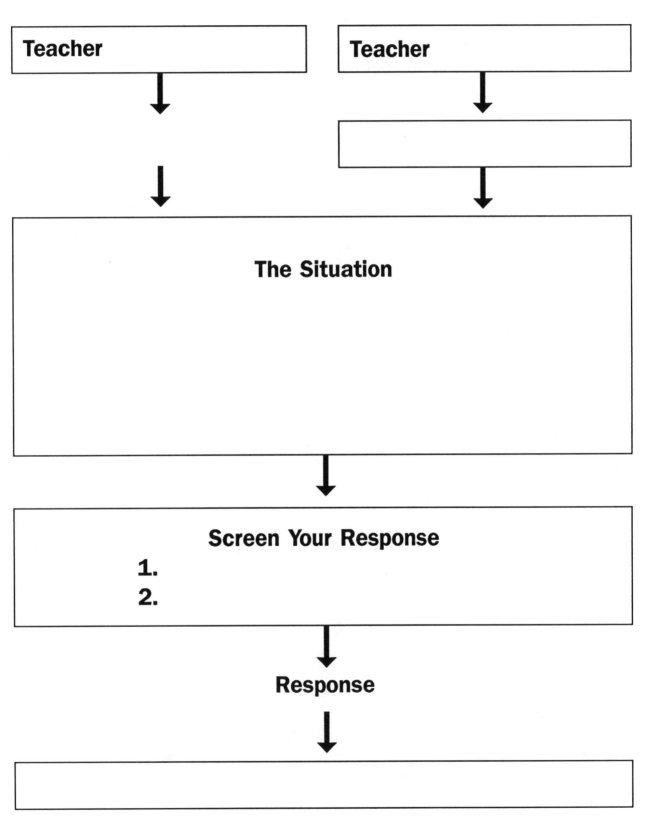

Teacher

Teacher

The Situation

Screen Your Response
1.
2.

Response

Overlay A

Assess

- **Relationship with Student/Parents**
- **Time and Place**
- **Student's Knowledge Base**
- **Student's Developmental Level**
- **Special Circumstances**

Real Question

| Teacher **Prepared** | Teacher **Surprised** |

Ask for more time

Assess
The Situation

- **Relationship with Student/Parents**
- **Time and Place**
- **Student's Knowledge Base**
- **Student's Developmental Level**
- **Special Circumstances**

Screen Your Response
1. *simple*
2. *encourage conversation*

Response

follow-up

CHAPTER 4

Methods for Early Elementary Grades

◆ OVERVIEW

Students are introduced to CDC's *Guidelines for Effective School Health Education to Prevent the Spread of AIDS* and to the other professional groups that contributed to the development of these guidelines. The students discuss essential HIV and AIDS content for early elementary grades provided in the guidelines. They then participate in learning opportunities that are appropriate for these grades. Finally, students brainstorm ways to integrate essential HIV and AIDS concepts into the early elementary curriculum.

◆ OBJECTIVES

- Students describe the purpose of the CDC's *Guidelines for Effective School Health Education to Prevent the Spread of AIDS*.
- Students describe and create developmentally appropriate learning opportunities for early elementary school children.

◆ MATERIALS

Transparency: **Consultants for CDC Guidelines**

Handout: **CDC Recommendations for HIV-Related Information Provided in Early Elementary Grades** (one for each student)

Supplies: One small container of glitter

Study prints, magazine or coloring book pictures, puppets, or books illustrating health helpers

Eight 9-inch round balloons

Dark, wide permanent marker (for writing on balloons)

Pillowcase or white kitchen trash bag labeled WORRIES

Straight pin

◆ ACTIVITIES

1. Explain that CDC has established guidelines that include essential HIV and AIDS information that will help children to avoid infection. Stress the word *essential*. Explain that the guidelines are intended to be a starting point, not an ending point, for education about HIV and AIDS.

Consultants for CDC Guidelines

American Academy of Pediatrics
American Association of School Administrators
American Public Health Association
American School Health Association
Association for the Advancement of Health Education
Association of State and Territorial Health Officers
Council of Chief State School Officers
National Congress of Parents and Teachers
National Council of Churches
National Education Association
National School Boards Association
Society of State Directors of Health, Physical Education, Recreation and Dance
U.S. Department of Education
U.S. Food and Drug Administration
U.S. Office of Disease Prevention and Health Promotion

Consultants for CDC Guidelines transparency

Show the **Consultants for CDC Guidelines** transparency to emphasize the high degree of expertise involved in the development of these guidelines.

Stress that the *Introduction* in the guidelines states that these guidelines "should not be construed as rules, but rather as a source of guidance." Point out that the guidelines also recommend that in the elementary grades "education about AIDS should be provided by the classroom teacher..." and that "the exact grades at which students receive information should be determined locally, in accord with community and parental values, and thus may vary from community to community."

2. Distribute the **CDC Recommendations for HIV-Related Information Provided in Early Elementary Grades** and identify the content considered to be essential for early elementary school children. Have students offer their opinions about the purpose of these guidelines.

3. Illustrate ways the essential content in the guidelines can be integrated into classroom lessons. Several demonstrations of learning opportunities for this level follow.

Education about HIV and AIDS can be integrated into a lesson on how germs spread.

- Use glitter to represent germs. Show how a handshake or a touch can transfer germs. Ask for suggestions of other substances that could be used to visualize the transfer of germs by touch (lipstick, flour, paint). Have your students name some diseases with which children are familiar such as the flu and chicken pox. List these diseases on the chalkboard.

- Following this demonstration, have students roleplay early elementary age children. Ask students, "Are *all* sicknesses caused by germs that are spread by touching?" (No.) Ask students to list some diseases that are spread in other ways. If AIDS is not mentioned, ask, "What is the new disease that is making some grown-ups very sick? Have you heard the name of the disease on the news?" Add AIDS to the list and continue adding other diseases. Be sure the list includes examples of communicable diseases. Briefly discuss each disease in terms of whether the diseases are spread by touching the sick person or touching items that have been used by the sick person. Explain that the developmental level of the children determines whether the term *communicable* is introduced.

- When the discussion reaches AIDS, provide the essential content identified in the CDC guidelines. Include the information that AIDS is caused by a germ (virus) called HIV.

- Remind students that by being sensitive to the reactions and concerns of the children, they can, as future teachers, determine whether additional information is needed. Point out that the end of the lesson would be an appropriate time to remind children that if they have questions about any sickness, they should ask an adult at home or school.

- Explain that this lesson could conclude with the children drawing faces showing how they feel when a friend is sick and pictures showing what they do to feel happy.

Education about HIV and AIDS can be integrated into a lesson on health helpers.

- Demonstrate how study prints, magazine or coloring book pictures, puppets, or books can be used to discuss health helpers who work to

CDC Recommendations for HIV-Related Information Provided in Early Elementary Grades handout

protect and promote our health. In the early elementary grades, children generally learn about police officers, firefighters, dentists, physicians, and nurses. They discuss these jobs and sometimes take field trips to see where these health helpers work. Riddles and charades are sometimes used to reinforce the lessons on health helpers.

- Tell students that *scientists* can be introduced as health helpers who use microscopes to see germs so small our eyes can't see them. Teachers can explain that by studying germs with the microscope, health helpers can learn how we can keep from getting sick.

- Point out that the introduction of scientists as health helpers provides a transition that allows teachers to ask, "What is the name of the new disease that scientists are studying? It is one that is making some grown-ups very sick."

Education about HIV and AIDS can be integrated into a mental health lesson.

Tell students to try the following exercises with the children they teach:

- Read aloud a story about a child who is worried about monsters in his closet and under his bed. Reassure children that occasional worries are a normal part of childhood. Explain that people of all ages have worries at times and that worries can be good when they cause us to be careful. Discuss the body's physical reactions to excessive worry (loss of appetite or gain in appetite, inability to sleep, rapid breathing, sweaty palms, irritability).

- Illustrate how too much worry can interfere with daily activities. Ask children to list common childhood worries (monsters, nobody likes me, lose my parent while shopping in a big store, sickness). As each worry is mentioned, blow up a balloon, write the worry on the balloon, show the children what you have written, and put the balloon into a pillowcase (or plastic trash bag) that is labeled WORRIES. If the children don't mention sickness as a worry, guide their discussion to include being sick. When the pillowcase is full of worries, hold the pillowcase and pantomime simple activities, such as coloring a picture, hugging someone, etc. Help children conclude that if we carry worries around with us, they interfere with daily activities.

- Lead the children in a discussion of ways that people can reduce or eliminate worries or fears. (They can talk about them. Get facts—sometimes we hear a scary noise and when we find out the cause of the noise, it isn't scary at all. Find out what others are doing about the problem. Ask for help. Find out what you can do to reduce the problem.)

- Bring the discussion back to the worry about being sick. Teachers could ask children what kinds of sickness cause worries and lead children to include AIDS in their list. Thus, the transition to HIV and AIDS-specific content has been made.

  Having mentioned AIDS, the teacher can identify AIDS as a disease caused by a germ (virus) called HIV. This germ is making some people feel very sick. Teachers should caution the children not to confuse the disease AIDS with school helpers called *aides* or with other synonyms or homonyms and reassure children. Specific examples of how HIV is *not* transmitted might be given. Teachers should stress that HIV is not caught from other children like a cold or the flu. More reassurance can be provided by reminding children that grown-ups have been told how to avoid HIV. Explain that people all over the world are learning about HIV and AIDS so they can stop the disease.

- After identifying the essential concepts in the CDC guidelines, answering children's questions, and covering appropriate information, teachers might direct attention back to *worry*. They can ask for ways that we could show care and concern for people who are worried or sick. The teacher might conclude the lesson by having children draw pictures for a bulletin board display of ways to show care and concern for others. Another way to conclude the lesson would be to have children roleplay ways to show care and concern.

4. Ask students to identify other areas of the early elementary curriculum into which education about HIV and AIDS might be integrated. Have students describe (orally or on paper) which demonstrations they might choose to use in their teaching. They should explain where the demonstration could be integrated into existing curricula.

Remind students that as teachers of early elementary school children they can contribute significantly to HIV prevention education by promoting self-esteem in young children and by providing basic concepts that will enable children to grasp more complex information as they progress to upper elementary grades.

Consultants for CDC Guidelines

American Academy of Pediatrics

American Association of School Administrators

American Public Health Association

American School Health Association

Association for the Advancement of Health Education

Association of State and Territorial Health Officers

Council of Chief State School Officers

National Congress of Parents and Teachers

National Council of Churches

National Education Association

National School Boards Association

Society of State Directors of Health, Physical Education, Recreation and Dance

U.S. Department of Education

U.S. Food and Drug Administration

U.S. Office of Disease Prevention and Health Promotion

CDC Recommendations for HIV-Related Information Provided in Elementary Grades

Content—General

Although information about the biology of the AIDS virus, the signs and symptoms of AIDS, and the social and economic costs of the epidemic might be of interest, such information is not the essential knowledge that students must acquire in order to prevent becoming infected with HIV. Similarly, a single film, lecture, or school assembly about AIDS will not be sufficient to assure that students develop the complex understanding and skills they will need to avoid becoming infected.

Schools should assure that students receive at least the essential information about AIDS, as summarized in sequence in the following pages, for each of three grade-level ranges. The exact grades at which students receive this essential information should be determined locally in accord with community and parental values, and thus may vary from community to community. Because essential information for students at higher grades requires an understanding of information essential for students at lower grades, secondary school personnel will need to assure that students understand basic concepts before teaching more advanced information. Schools simultaneously should assure that students have opportunities to learn about emotional and social factors that influence types of behavior associated with HIV transmission.

Early Elementary School

Education about AIDS for students in early elementary grades principally should be designed to allay excessive fears of the epidemic and of becoming infected.

- *AIDS is a disease that is causing some adults to get very sick, but it does not commonly affect children.*
- *You do not get AIDS just by being near or touching someone who has it.*
- *Scientists all over the world are working hard to find a way to stop people from getting AIDS and to cure those who have it.*

Centers for Disease Control. Guidelines for Effective School Health Education to Prevent the Spread of AIDS. *MMWR* 1988; 37 (suppl. no. S-2): page 5. Revised by D. Peter Drotman, MD. Centers for Disease Control, Center for Infectious Diseases, Division of HIV/AIDS. 1991.

CHAPTER 5 Methods for Late Elementary/Middle School Grades

◆ OVERVIEW

Students discuss characteristics of children in late elementary/middle school grades and examine **CDC Recommendations for HIV-Related Information Provided in Late Elementary/Middle School Grades**. Then students participate in demonstrations of learning opportunities for these grade levels. Appropriate content for HIV prevention education is illustrated in the demonstrations. Students then explore issues related to teaching about sexual transmission of HIV.

◆ OBJECTIVES

- Students correlate developmental characteristics of children in the fourth through eighth grades with the essential information for HIV prevention education.

- Students describe appropriate strategies to teach children in upper elementary grades about HIV and AIDS.

◆ MATERIALS

Handout: **CDC Recommendations for HIV-Related Information Provided in Late Elementary/Middle School Grades** (one for each student)

Supplies: Tennis ball

Golf ball

Miniature marshmallow

Large plastic egg (such as L'eggs egg) that splits into halves

Ten to fifteen small marshmallows

Two clear, plastic bottles (juice bottles, tennis ball cans, or peanut butter jars) without labels, one half-filled with pale green water and the other half-filled with dark red water

Tape

Two pencils

Two small toys

Large see-through baster

Rag

Ten large pictures of men and women from various age and racial groups; include pictures of individuals living in city, suburban, and rural environments

◆ ACTIVITIES

1. Review the developmental characteristics of children in upper elementary grades. Begin a discussion about the appropriate focus of methodology for education about AIDS and HIV at this level. Use the following points to frame the discussion and review:

   • In the late elementary grades, children have become more social with peers, and they are dealing with an emerging sense of their own sexuality. They are less open with their parents and often become more private and withdrawn. Typically, they are more embarrassed by sexual questions. They are approaching, or may have reached, their first real-life encounter with pressures to participate in sexual or drug-related activities.

   • Children in the late elementary grades are at the threshold of adolescence. Based on the following profile, a 9- or 10-year-old child should receive short, multiple lessons about HIV and AIDS.

I. **Continues to:**
- think and act concretely
- play children's games
- enjoy the intimacy of family

II. **Beginning to:**
- think and act abstractly
- pay greater attention to styles of dress, dance and music
- distance from the family

III. **Develops:**
- cognitive understanding of cause-and-effect relationships
- tolerance of ambiguity and less insistence on black-and-white solutions
- an understanding of the variety of human sexual activities and the consequences of sexual behavior (unwanted pregnancies, STDs)
- a concern for the welfare of others
- a growing interest in community values ◇◇

◇◇Source: Quackenbush, M. and S. Villarreal. 1988. *"Does AIDS Hurt?"* Santa Cruz, Calif.: ETR Associates.

Nine to ten years is the time to move from the early elementary focus on "what HIV and AIDS aren't" to a direct focus on "what HIV and AIDS are." Children of this age are characteristically curious and daring, and they have a strong sense of immortality. Children in this age group must be introduced to their own vulnerability to HIV infection. Teachers can help them internalize a sense of vulnerability by identifying the extent of the problem—locally, nationally, and worldwide. To make HIV and AIDS seem less remote and distant, teachers may invite guest speakers and assign readings or interviews that help children comprehend the impact of HIV infection on the lives of infected individuals, and on families and friends.

Children who may never be at high risk for HIV infection need to be aware of the impact of AIDS on the entire social and medical care systems in our nation, so they do not become complacent in their response to the AIDS crisis, seeing it as somebody else's problem.

- Fear can have a paralyzing effect; women may fear cancer so strongly that they refuse to do breast self-examinations. We must, therefore, balance children's feelings of vulnerability with a feeling of control over the situation. Children can gain this sense of control by acquiring specific knowledge and skills. This knowledge includes how HIV affects the immune system, how it is transmitted, and how it can be prevented. The skills needed are skills in communicating, decision making, and resisting peer pressure.

- Needed skills are not specific to education about HIV and AIDS. Skill-building in communication, decision making and saying no are components of many school programs. An effective way to present specific information is through the use of audio-visual materials. However, all materials must be carefully screened. Some are inaccurate, some are too graphic or too explicit for young audiences, and some, in presuming a sexually active audience, may seem to imply that sexual activity in upper elementary grades is normal behavior rather than an exception. Programs designed for public television stations (instructional television) and for commercial television should not be overlooked. They may be appropriate, as well as cost effective. School policies can provide guidance in media selection and use.

- Demonstrations, skits, bulletin boards, research reports, group activities, and other methods can all be used to present HIV-specific information. Activities such as brainstorming and non-guided discussion are only appropriate for certain aspects of education about HIV and AIDS. It is not recommended, for example, that a teacher have children brainstorm ways that people transmit HIV, because this method jeopardizes control of a sensitive discussion. Most schools have policies or standards that identify the parameters for a discussion of sexual intercourse and alternate sexual lifestyles. Saying "the discussion got out of hand" is not an acceptable response from a teacher who allows a discussion to cross the boundaries established by the school and community.

2. Distribute the **CDC Recommendations for HIV-Related Information Provided in Late Elementary/Middle School Grades** and review the content. Remind students that the content identified on the handout is suggested as *essential* content. Education about HIV and AIDS is not to be limited to content in the CDC guidelines.

3. Illustrate ways that teachers might present HIV-specific content in late elementary and middle school grades. Several demonstrations of learning opportunities appropriate for this level follow.

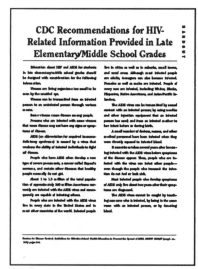

CDC Recommendations for HIV-Related Information Provided in Late Elementary/Middle School Grades handout

Use a video to present essential content about the immune system.

- Children do not have to understand how the immune system functions and what T-cells do, but they do need to understand that HIV weakens a person's ability to fight off disease. Several educational videos are available for use in teaching about the function of the immune system. Two that are recommended are "The Immune System: Your Magic Doctor," by Barr Films, 12801 Schabarum Ave., P.O. Box 7878, Irwindale, CA 91706-7878, (800) 234-7878, and "Slim Goodbody: AIDS and the Immune System," available from the Agency for Instructional Television, 111 W. 17th St., Bloomington, IN 47401, (800) 477-4509.

- With knowledge of the immune system, children can understand what is meant when we say that the AIDS virus, called HIV (human immunodeficiency virus), cripples the immune system.

- Explain that HIV destroys the "control centers" (certain white blood cells, called T-helper cells) of the immune system. When this happens the body cannot properly defend itself against certain infections and other diseases. Explain that the person with AIDS does not usually die of HIV infection directly—the person with AIDS usually dies from other diseases that the immune system cannot fight off. Most often, the person with AIDS dies from a type of rare pneumonia or a cancer called Kaposi's sarcoma.

- Have students brainstorm other activities for children that would show their understanding of the immune system.

Show how teachers can help children visualize the size of viruses.

- To illustrate the small size of germs, show the students a tennis ball, a golf ball, and a miniature marshmallow. Explain that if we use the tennis and golf balls to represent the range of sizes of bacteria, then the marshmallow would represent the size of the HIV virus. Suggest that as an art integration activity teachers might have children draw their interpretations of bacteria and viruses for a bulletin board display.

Demonstrate how viruses invade and destroy cells.

- Explain that viruses are not cells. They are germs that cannot reproduce themselves. They have to enter a cell in order to complete their life cycles.

- Hold up a large plastic egg that has ten to fifteen small marshmallows slipped into it (unknown to students) and explain that this egg represents a cell. Use one marshmallow to represent a virus. Put the "virus" into the "cell" as you explain that viruses take over a cell and cause it to reproduce viruses instead of carrying out the cell's usual function. After viruses reproduce in a living cell, they escape from it by bursting out. This can kill the cell. Pull apart the halves of the egg to show the small marshmallows flying out, demonstrating how new viruses are scattered about to find, infect, and multiply in other cells.

- Conclude the demonstration by reminding students that HIV, the virus that causes AIDS, infects and destroys white blood cells (T-helper cells, primarily) that direct the immune system's battle against infections and disease. Holding the two halves of the egg, explain that the white blood cells that help fight disease and infections are destroyed.

Demonstrate the concept that HIV is not spread through casual contact.

- Display two clear plastic bottles, one half-filled with dark red water and the other with pale green water. Explain that the bottles represent our bodies' skin, representing the boundary between our bodies and outside elements. Show that holding the bottles (bodies) near each other does not cause mixing of the colored fluids—nor does rubbing or bumping the bottles together.

- Using tape, attach a pencil to each container. Demonstrate that trading pencils does not cause the colored fluids to be exchanged. Repeat the demonstration with small toys.

- Explain that HIV must enter the body of a person in order to cause HIV infection.

Demonstrate how needles and syringes can spread HIV.

- Using a kitchen baster, withdraw some red fluid from the bottle to demonstrate how HIV-infected blood can be drawn into a syringe and remain to infect another person who might use the same syringe. Squeeze out the fluid, wipe off the outside of the baster and show the red droplets that are still visible on the inside. Conclude that carefully wiping a needle and syringe does not remove HIV.

Illustrate that people who are infected with HIV may not have any signs or symptoms and that HIV-infected people include all races, both sexes, and all ages.

- Show magazine pictures, suggesting that groups of children could be asked to rank them from the most likely to be HIV-infected to the least likely to be HIV-infected. In discussing reasons for group opinions, teachers should identify and correct misinformation about HIV infection. They should stress that one cannot tell by looking at people whether they are HIV-infected, and that people who are infected with HIV live in every state in the United States and in most other countries of the world. Point out that infected people live in cities as well as in suburbs, small towns, and rural areas. Most infected people are adults, but a growing number of teenagers are becoming infected. Women and men of every race are infected, including Asian/Pacific Islanders, Native Americans, African-Americans, Whites, and Latinos.

Discuss how HIV is spreading rapidly and is one of the most serious health problems that the world is now facing.

- Explain that thousands of people have already died as a result of AIDS, and approximately one million Americans are HIV-infected and capable of infecting others. Children often have difficulty comprehending large numbers. Ask students to determine the distance that 1 million people would cover if they stood arm-in-arm (allowing two feet per person). They should find that distance to be 378.78 miles. The distance of 379 miles may be meaningless to children until they identify a familiar point 379 miles away from their school or home.

- Ask, "If all the HIV-infected people in the United States stood arm-in-arm along an expressway, how long would it take to drive from the first person to the last at a speed of 60 miles per hour?" (Answer: about 6 hours and 20 minutes—if we don't stop for any breaks.)

- Ask students to brainstorm suggestions for other ways that this statistic might be simplified for children's understanding.

- Suggest that children could work in cooperative learning groups to write and present skits showing the extent of the AIDS epidemic. These might take the form of interviews with scientists or health care workers.

4. Remind students that HIV is spread by sexual intercourse and reusing IV drug needles. HIV is present in blood, semen, and vaginal fluids.

If a school provides lessons on human reproduction, children in the middle elementary school grades will likely already have a working definition of semen, vaginal fluid, and sexual intercourse. The classroom teacher can identify semen and vaginal fluids as fluids that can transmit HIV to the bloodstream of a partner during sexual intercourse.

The classroom teacher can simply identify *semen* and *vaginal fluids* as fluids that can contain HIV. HIV can be transmitted to a partner during sexual activity. HIV enters through tiny, perhaps invisible, breaks in the skin or mucous membranes that line the mouth, vagina, and rectum.

If children have not had lessons on human reproduction, or if school policy does not permit sexual intercourse to be fully explained, school policy may permit teachers to say that "when a man and a woman have sexual intercourse, semen from the man travels through his penis into the woman's vagina, and then sperm can move to join with an egg in the woman and start the growth of a baby."

It is important that upper elementary and middle school students understand that when blood, semen, or vaginal fluids *from an HIV-infected person* enters another person, infection often occurs.

5. Acknowledge that human breast milk is believed to transmit HIV to babies, but only a few instances worldwide substantiate this.

6. After identifying blood, vaginal fluids, and semen as fluids that transmit HIV, recommend that *abstinence from sex and intravenous drug use are the most effective methods of prevention.*

    If school policy recommends that information on condom use be presented to upper elementary grade or middle school students, instruct children on how to use condoms correctly. Information on the failure rate of condoms should also be included. Presenting condom use as if it were as effective as abstinence at preventing HIV transmission is inappropriate. Education to prevent intercourse is preferred to education to prevent HIV transmission during intercourse, especially for elementary age children.

    Other concepts related to prevention include taking responsibility for your own health and the health of others, the decision-making process, and how to say no to peer pressure.

7. The examples provided in this chapter show how education about HIV and AIDS can be presented through a variety of learning experiences. Have students describe places in the upper elementary school curriculum where specific HIV and AIDS activities could be appropriately incorporated.

CDC Recommendations for HIV-Related Information Provided in Late Elementary/Middle School Grades

Education about HIV and AIDS for students in late elementary/middle school grades should be designed with consideration for the following information.

Viruses are living organisms too small to be seen by the unaided eye.

Viruses can be transmitted from an infected person to an uninfected person through various means.

Some viruses cause disease among people.

Persons who are infected with some viruses that cause disease may not have any signs or symptoms of disease.

AIDS (an abbreviation for acquired immunodeficiency syndrome) is caused by a virus that weakens the ability of infected individuals to fight off disease.

People who have AIDS often develop a rare type of severe pneumonia, a cancer called Kaposi's sarcoma, and certain other diseases that healthy people normally do not get.

About 1 to 1.5 million of the total population of approximately 240 million Americans currently are infected with the AIDS virus and consequently are capable of infecting others.

People who are infected with the AIDS virus live in every state in the United States and in most other countries of the world. Infected people live in cities as well as in suburbs, small towns, and rural areas. Although most infected people are adults, teenagers can also become infected. Females as well as males are infected. People of every race are infected, including Whites, Blacks, Hispanics, Native Americans, and Asian/Pacific Islanders.

The AIDS virus can be transmitted by sexual contact with an infected person; by using needles and other injection equipment that an infected person has used; and from an infected mother to her infant before or during birth.

A small number of doctors, nurses, and other medical personnel have been infected when they were directly exposed to infected blood.

It sometimes takes several years after becoming infected with the AIDS virus before symptoms of the disease appear. Thus, people who are infected with the virus can infect other people—even though the people who transmit the infection do not feel or look sick.

Most infected people who develop symptoms of AIDS only live about two years after their symptoms are diagnosed.

The AIDS virus cannot be caught by touching someone who is infected, by being in the same room with an infected person, or by donating blood.

Centers for Disease Control. Guidelines for Effective School Health Education to Prevent the Spread of AIDS. *MMWR* 1988;37 (suppl. no. S-2): pages 5-6.

CHAPTER 6
Reassessing Personal Feelings and Staying Informed

♦ **OVERVIEW**

Students reexamine their feelings about teaching HIV prevention and AIDS information. They discuss issues of concern and ways to keep HIV information updated. Students begin an outside assignment on designing strategies for HIV prevention education.

♦ **OBJECTIVES**

- Students describe the importance of a positive attitude toward HIV prevention education in the elementary and middle school grades.
- Students identify reliable sources of current information on HIV and AIDS.
- Students design an appropriate strategy for presenting HIV-specific information to elementary and middle school students (grades kindergarten through eighth).

◆ MATERIALS

Handout: **Why Elementary/Middle School Teachers Might Choose *Not* to Teach About HIV and AIDS** (completed by each student in Chapter 1)

Handout: **HIV Prevention Assignment** (one for each student)

◆ ACTIVITIES

1. Have students examine their earlier responses on the handout **Why Elementary/Middle School Teachers Might Choose *Not* to Teach About HIV and AIDS** (completed in Chapter 1). Ask them to indicate any changes in their feelings by drawing boxes around responses they would choose now.

   Invite volunteers to describe changes that have occurred. Collect and review this handout. Provide counsel for students whose responses reflect discomfort with HIV prevention education.

2. Education about HIV and AIDS is not easy. Although any teacher can teach about the disease, the challenge is to strengthen the teacher's level of comfort with sensitive issues associated with the subject. An open discussion of the issues is one way to add to this level of comfort.

   Lead a discussion about issues still of concern to your students. Encourage all students to participate. Present each of the following issues one at a time. Have students consider each issue mentally or in writing before holding a whole-class discussion. The *Discussion* sections that follow the listed issues are provided for background and not intended as lectures.

   Issue: *I think I will be uncomfortable teaching about HIV and AIDS.*
   Discussion: Teaching about HIV and AIDS can be uncomfortable, especially in a teacher's first attempt with material. A familiarity with content, a plan for answering student questions, a familiarity with school and district guidelines, and a willingness to consider both sides of an issue help combat discomfort.
   Because of the sensitivity of HIV prevention education issues and because different children are more comfortable with different teachers, one way to ensure that children's needs are being met is to team

Why Elementary/Middle
School Teachers Might
Choose *Not* to Teach
About HIV and AIDS
handout

teach. A child may make a comment to one teacher that he or she would not make to the other. Various teaching styles may draw out different children in different ways at different times.

Team teaching or using guest speakers can provide a temporary solution until the teacher has received whatever additional preparation is warranted. Building a sense of comfort with HIV information is essential, however, because teachers deal with children on a daily basis, answering spontaneous questions and hearing student concerns.

Future teachers may want to consider additional courses of study, such as sex education, death education, and drug education courses.

Issue: *It's not a problem in my town.*

Discussion: AIDS is a worldwide problem. Contacting a local HIV and AIDS task force may be useful in identifying the extent of the local problem. However, whether or not HIV infection is a major local problem, the mobility of today's population and the social, economic, medical, and personal issues of HIV and AIDS combine to create a situation with which all people should be concerned.

Issue: *Kids have no interest in HIV and AIDS. Why give them something to worry about?*

Discussion: Children whose lives have not yet been touched by the AIDS epidemic probably do not have major concerns related to this topic. However, children who have heard about this "killer disease" from television or adult conversations may have fears, questions, or misinformation that, once addressed, will eliminate needless worry, not create worry. A major goal of education about HIV and AIDS for the young child is to eliminate fears and worries.

Issue: *There is no room in my full schedule to include lessons on HIV and AIDS.*

Discussion: HIV prevention education correlates and/or integrates easily into traditional elementary and middle school curricula. Time spent reducing fears and addressing children's concerns about their own health and well-being or the health and well-being of loved ones frees children to give full attention to other demands of learning.

In late elementary and middle school, several lessons might be required to adequately cover HIV-specific lessons. This material correlates with other health topics, such as disease, body systems, drug abuse, compassion for the sick, community health issues, decision making, and self-esteem.

At the end of the whole-class discussion, ask students to review all the issues and make some generalizations that summarize their feelings and attitudes. Summaries should include an explanation of the importance of a positive teacher attitude as a component of HIV prevention education.

3. Direct the students' attention to the **Essential Readings** and **HIV/AIDS Education Resources** in the appendix. Remind them that, in addition to materials suggested here for further reading, periodic updates on HIV and AIDS information are available from a variety of resources.

    Discuss the purpose of AIDS hotlines and remind students that most communities are developing HIV prevention education resources. Remind them that professional health organizations are also excellent resources for updating information. Two other reliable sources of information are the local and state departments of health.

4. Distribute the **HIV Prevention Assignment** about designing strategies for HIV prevention education and explain the assignment to your students.

HIV Prevention Assignment handout

HIV Prevention Assignment

Part A – Questions to Consider

Write a response that you feel would be appropriate in a classroom setting for the question "How do people get AIDS?" for each situation described below.

1. A kindergarten child with no previous classroom discussion of AIDS.

2. A second grade child who has learned that germs cause sickness and who has heard on TV that people are dying of a serious disease called AIDS.

3. A fifth grade child whose parents have clearly opposed sex education for their children.

4. A fifth grade child who has completed a K-5 sex education program.

Part B – Create a Stategy

Create one strategy for presenting HIV-specific information to elementary school students. This strategy must be fully developed and may take the form of a demonstration, a skit, a group activity, or other appropriate method of teaching. The teaching strategy must include appropriate follow-up discussion questions (and desired responses). The grade level, number of students, setting, and any special circumstances (e.g., special-needs children) are to be identified.

Essential Readings

A unified approach to health teaching. 1983. Position statement. Reston, Va: Association for the Advancement of Health Education.

AIDS. 1989. (Special issue.) *Health Education* 19, no. 6.

AIDS/HIV Infection Education. 1988. (Special issue.) *Journal of School Health* 58, no. 8:1.

AIDS: Are children at risk? 1986. Washington, D.C.: American Association of Colleges for Teacher Education. (ERIC Document Reproduction Service. Fact Sheet No. 16.)

Being at ease with handicapped children. 1984. Reston, Va: Clearinghouse on Handicapped and Gifted Children. (ERIC Document Reproduction Service.)

Brown, L. K. and G. K. Fritz. 1988. AIDS education in the schools: A literature review as a guide for curriculum planning. *Clinical Pediatrics* 27:311-16.

Burnette, J. 1987. *Adapting instructional materials for mainstreamed students* (contract No. 400-84-0010). Reston, Va: The Council for Exceptional Children.

Centers for Disease Control. 1988. Guidelines for effective school health education to prevent the spread of AIDS. *Morbidity and Mortality Weekly Report* 37(S-2). Atlanta, Ga: Centers for Disease Control.

Coalition of National Health Education Organizations. 1988. *Instruction about AIDS within the school curriculum*. Position paper. New York: National Center for Health Education.

Cortese, P., R. Everst, W. Jubb, C. Nickerson, M. Pollock, B. Simon and M. Wantz. 1984. *Comprehensive school health education*. The National Comprehensive School Health Education Guidelines Committee. Reston, Va: Association for the Advancement of Health Education.

Criteria for evaluating an AIDS curriculum. 1988. Boston: National Coalition of Advocates for Students.

DiClemente, R. J., C. B. Boyer and E. S. Morales. 1988. Minorities and AIDS:

Knowledge, attitudes and misconceptions among Black and Latino adolescents. *Public Health Briefs* 78:55-57.

Disabilities: An overview. 1987. Reston, Va: Clearinghouse on Handicapped and Gifted Children. (ERIC Document Reproduction Service. Fact Sheet No. 420.)

Fineberg, H. V. 1988. Education to prevent AIDS: Prospects and obstacles. *Science* 239(4840): 592-596.

Fineberg, H. V. 1988. The social dimensions of AIDS. *Scientific American* 259(October): 118-134.

Heyward, W. L. and I. W. Curran. 1988. The epidemiology of AIDS in the U.S. *Scientific American* 259(October): 72-81.

Lifson, A. R. 1988. Do alternative modes for transmission of human immunodeficiency virus exist? *Journal of the American Medical Association* 259(9): 1353-1356.

Luty, E. T. 1988. Controversial topics in a health education program. *Health Education* E:39-44.

Kolbe, L., J. Jones, G. Nelson, L. Daily, C. Duncan, L. Kann, A. Lawrence, B. Broyles and D. Poehler. 1988. School health education to prevent the spread of AIDS: Overview of a national program. *Hygiene* 7(3): 10-13.

Managing communicable and contagious diseases. Policy statement. Reston, Va: The Council for Exceptional Children.

Quackenbush, M. and S. Villeareal. 1988. *"Does Aids Hurt?" Educating Young Children About AIDS*. Santa Cruz, Calif.: ETR Associates.

Steps to help your school set up an AIDS education program. 1988. Boston: National Coalition of Advocates for Students.

Tolsma, D. 1988. Activities of the Centers for Disease Control in AIDS education. *Journal of School Health* 58(4): 133-136.

Turner, N. H., J. McLaughlin and J. C. Shruh. 1988. AIDS education: Process, content, and strategies. *Health Values* 12:6-12.

United States Department of Health and Human Services. Public Health Service. Centers for Disease Control. Office of the Deputy Director (AIDS). 1988. *AIDS and Minorities*. Washington, D.C.: National Conference on the Prevention of HIV Infection and AIDS among Racial and Ethnic Minorities in the United States.

Walters, L. 1988. Ethical issues in the prevention and treatment of HIV infection and AIDS. *Science* 239(4840): 597-603.

HIV/AIDS Education Resources

Several national resources are available to assist teachers in presenting HIV/AIDS education. These resources can provide current information about the HIV epidemic, educational materials, and teaching strategies. A few national organizations publish journals or newsletters that often list current materials and professional preparatory opportunities that offer articles about HIV infection.

In addition to your state or local health departments, the following resources may be useful:

National Hotlines

National AIDS Information Line
(800) 342-AIDS (English-speaking)
(800) 344-SIDA (Spanish-speaking)
(800) AIDSTTY (hearing-impaired)

National Institute on Drug Abuse
Drug Abuse Treatment Information and Referral Line
(800) 662-HELP

National Institutes of Health
National Institute of Allergy and Infectious Diseases (NIAID)
(Information on experimental therapies for AIDS and HIV infection)
(800) TRIALS-A

National Gay and Lesbian Crisis Line
(800) 767-4297

National Clearinghouse

National AIDS Information Clearinghouse
P.O. Box 6003
Rockville, MD 20850
(800) 458-5231

Computerized Bibliographic Database

AIDS School Health Education Subfile on the Combined Health Information Database (CHID)

Contains programs and curricula; health policies, regulations and guidelines; and materials for schools. Managed by the U.S. Public Health Service.

BRS Information Technologies
Div. of Maxwell Online
1200 Route 7
Latham, NY 12110
(800) 289-4277

National Organizations

American Association of School Administrators
Office of Minority Affairs -- AIDS
1801 North Moore Street
Arlington, VA 22209
(703) 528-0700

American College Health Association
1300 Piccard Drive, Suite 200
Rockville, MD 20850
(301) 963-1100

American Federation of Teachers
555 New Jersey Avenue NW
Washington, DC 20001
(202) 879-4548

American Foundation for AIDS Research
(The AIDS Information Resources Directory)
1515 Broadway, Suite 3601
New York, NY 10036
(212) 719-0033

American Medical Association
Office of HIV
515 North State Street
Chicago, IL 60610
(312) 464-4566

American Red Cross
Office of HIV/AIDS Education
1709 New York Avenue NW, Suite 208
Washington, DC 20006
(202) 434-4077

American School Health Association
(Journal: *Journal of School Health*)
P.O. Box 708
Kent, OH 44240
(216) 678-1601

Association for the Advancement of Health Education
An Association of the American Alliance for Health, Physical Education, Recreation, and Dance
(Journal: *Health Education*)
1900 Association Drive
Reston, VA 22091
(703) 476-3437

Center for Population Options
1025 Vermont Avenue NW, Suite 210
Washington, DC 20005
(202) 347-5700

Council of Chief State School Officers
Resource Center on Educational Inquiry
400 North Capitol Street NW, Suite 379
Washington, DC 20001
(202) 393-8159

ETR Associates
(Catalog on AIDS and Family Life Education Materials; Journal: *Family Life Educator*)
P.O. Box 1830
Santa Cruz, CA 95061-1830
(800) 321-4407

Hispanic AIDS Forum
121 Avenue of the Americas, Suite 505
New York, NY 10013
(212) 966-6336

Minority Task Force on AIDS
National Council of Churches
475 Riverside Drive, Room 572
New York, NY 10115
(212) 870-2385

National Association of People with AIDS
P. O. Box 18345
Washington, DC 20036
(202) 429-2856

National Association of State Boards of
    Education
1012 Cameron Street
Alexandria, VA 22314
(703) 684-4000

National Coalition of Advocates for Students
100 Boylston Street, Suite 737
Boston, MA 02116-4610
(617) 357-8507

National Coalition of Hispanic Health and
    Human Services Organizations
1030 15th Street NW, Suite 1053
Washington, DC 20005
(202) 371-2100

National Commission on Correctional
    Health Care
2105 N. South Port, Suite 200
Chicago, IL 60614
(312) 528-0818

National Education Association (NEA)
1590 Adamson Parkway, Suite 260
Morrow, GA 30260
(404) 960-1325

National Network of Runaways and Youth
    Services, Inc.
1400 Eye Street NW, Suite 330
Washington, DC 20005
(202) 682-4114

National Organization of Black County
    Officials
440 First Street NW, Suite 500
Washington, DC 20001
(202) 347-6953

The National PTA
700 North Rush Street
Chicago, IL 60611
(312) 787-0977

National Rural and Small School Consortium
National Rural Development Institute
Miller Hall 359
Western Washington University
Bellingham, WA 98225
(206) 676-3576

National School Boards Association
1680 Duke Street
Alexandria, VA 22314
(703) 838-6756

San Francisco AIDS Foundation
(AIDS Educator: *A Catalog of AIDS
    Educational Material*)
P. O. Box 6182
San Francisco, CA 94101-6182
(415) 864-5855; (800) 863-2437

Newsletters

AIDS Alert
American Health Consultants
67 Peachtree Park Drive, NE
Atlanta, GA 30309
(404) 351-4523

The AIDS/HIV Record
BIODATA Publishers
P.O. Box 66020
Washington, DC 20035-6020
(202) 393-AIDS

AIDS Literature & News Review
University Publishing Group
107 East Church Street
Frederick, MD 21701
(800) 654-8188

AIDS Targeted Information Newsletter
Williams & Wilkins
428 E. Preston Street
Baltimore, MD 21202
(800) 638-6423

Morbidity and Mortality Weekly Report
National AIDS Information Clearinghouse
P.O. Box 6003
Rockville, MD 20850
(301) 251-5642

SIECUS Report
Sex Information and Education Council of
    the United States (SIECUS)
130 West 42nd Street, 25th Floor
New York, NY 10036
(212) 819-9770